Weird Facts about Food (Gross.)

Disgusting (but True!) Food Trivia to Shock Your Friends and Ruin Snack Time

Pamela Pettyfeather

PETTYFEATHER
PUBLISHING

Contents

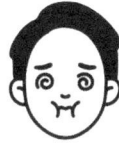

INTRODUCTION:
What's in Your Mouth?

Hey.

Quick question: **Do you know what you're eating right now?** Like, *really* know?

Because that "natural flavor" in your juice might come from a **beaver's butt gland**. That gummy bear? It's held together with **boiled cow skin**. And that red candy? Mmm... **crushed beetle juice.** Sweet. Still hungry?

If you love fun facts, gross stuff, weird science, and surprising history, you're in the right place. This book is jam-packed with:

- **True trivia** that sounds fake

- **Actual foods** people eat every day (and some they really shouldn't)

- **Stomach-churning** ingredients hiding in plain sight

- And **horrifying discoveries** that will make you say: "Wait—WHAT?!"

We're talking about **maggot cheese, toe cheese**, and **cheese that isn't even cheese**. We'll meet exploding octopus tentacles, burping bacteria, and brain-melting meat glue.

This book isn't here to ruin food forever...

(Okay, maybe a little.)

It's here to help you:

- Look closer

- Ask better questions

- Win arguments with your friends

- And become the **grossest, smartest person at the dinner table**

So if you're ready to laugh, gag, learn something weird, and ruin dessert for everyone... LET'S DIG IN. ☺

Chapter 1

Hidden Horrors in Everyday Foods

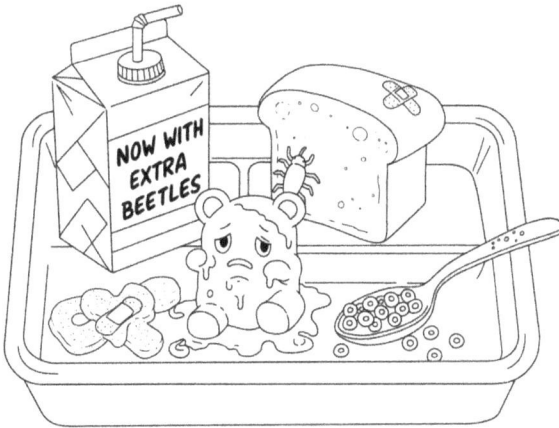

You probably think you know what's in your favorite foods. Chocolate? Delicious. Bread? Fluffy goodness. But guess what? Some of your everyday snacks are hiding **secret**

ingredients that are seriously **gross**. Ready to ruin snack time?

Let's go.

~

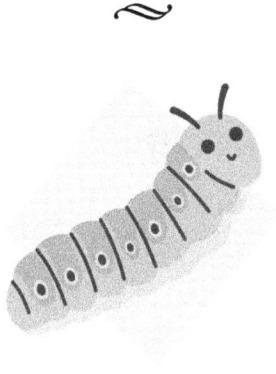

1. Crushed Bugs in Your Juice and Candy
1. Crushed Bugs in Your Juice and Candy

Gross Meter: 💀💀💀

That shiny red color in strawberry yogurt, pink lemonade, or red jelly beans? It might come from a little something called **cochineal extract**—a dye made by **crushing tiny beetles** that live on cactus plants. The bugs are boiled, dried, and ground up to create a bright red color.

It's totally natural. It's also **literally bug guts**.

2. Vanilla Flavoring... From a Beaver's Butt

Gross Meter: 💀💀💀💀

Vanilla ice cream is made with vanilla beans... right?

Sometimes. "Natural flavoring" in vanilla products **can also come from castoreum**, a gooey substance produced by

glands near a beaver's butt. Castoreum smells like vanilla and has been used in perfumes and food for decades.

But you won't see "beaver gland juice" on the label—it'll just say **"natural flavor."** Appetizing! (But lucky you–because of advances in synthetic vanilla flavor development, castoreum is not as common in foods as it used to be.)

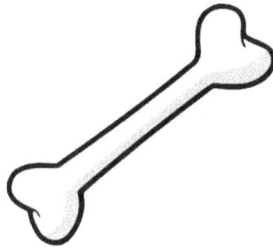

3. Gummy Bears = Animal Bones

Gross Meter: 🤮🤮

What gives gummies that perfect bounce?

Gelatin. It's made by boiling down **pig skin, cow bones, and animal tendons** into a thick goo that solidifies into chewy treats. It's also in marshmallows, Jell-O, and some frosted cereals.

Next time you chomp a gummy worm, remember: That squishy snack used to be somebody's *leg*.

4. Human Hair in Your Bread Dough

Gross Meter: 🤢👻

Some commercial bread dough includes an ingredient called **L-cysteine**, which makes bread softer and fluffier. Sounds harmless—until you learn that L-cysteine can be made from **duck feathers**... or **human hair** (often collected from barber shops in China).

That croissant you love? Might just have a little off-the-top baked in. ✂️

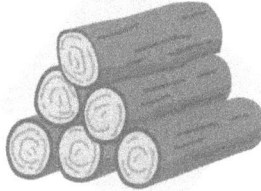

5. Wood Pulp in Shredded Cheese

Gross Meter: 🤢

You know that fluffy coating that keeps shredded cheese from clumping? That's **cellulose**—which is made from **wood pulp**.

Yep. You're eating powdered trees.

It's totally legal, safe to eat, and even FDA-approved. But still—sawdust tacos, anyone?

6. Firefighting Foam in Soda?

Gross Meter: ☺

Some fizzy drinks use an ingredient called **brominated vegetable oil (BVO)**. It keeps flavor evenly mixed... but it's also used in **flame retardants**. Too much BVO has been linked to memory loss and skin problems. It's banned in Europe and Japan.

Still allowed in U.S. sodas, though (until August 2025)! ☺

GROSS ORIGINS

QUIZ

Match the ingredient to what it's made from:

A) Gelatin   1) Crushed bugs

B) Cochineal   2) Pig bones

C) Cellulose   3) Beaver butt glands

D) L-cysteine   4) Human hair

E) Castoreum   5) Wood pulp

GROSS!

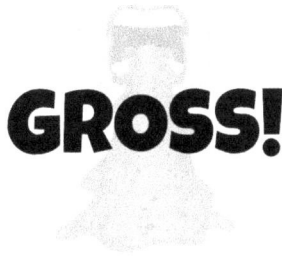

Chapter Recap: What Did You Just Eat?!

If you've ever had:

- Fruit punch

- Marshmallows

- Gummy bears

- Cheddar cheese

- A frosted doughnut

... Congratulations!

You may have swallowed **bugs**, **bones**, **beaver butt juice**, or **hair**—and didn't even know it. Welcome to the weird world of food science.

Up next: Get ready to time travel to the **grossest recipes in history**, from moldy fish sauce to candy made with poison.

Chapter 2

Rotten, Rancid, and Really Old Recipes

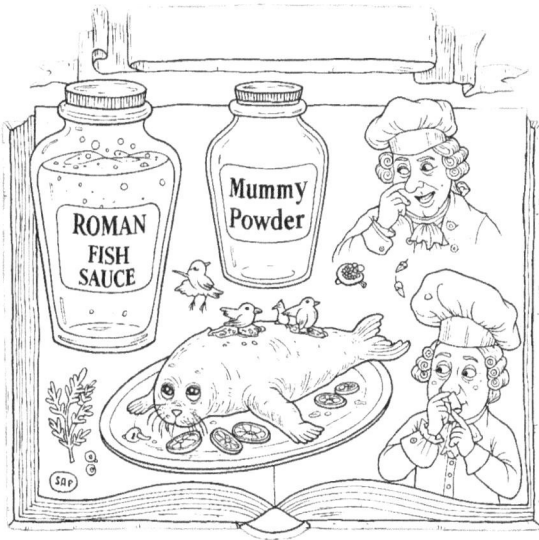

Think today's food is weird?

Wait until you see what people used to eat **on purpose**. From fermented fish guts to poisonous candy, the past is packed with **questionable cuisine** that would send modern food inspectors running for the hills.

Let's open the ancient cookbook and see what's for dinner!

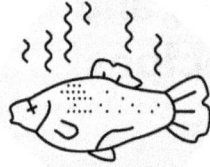

~

1. Ancient Rome's Favorite Condiment? Rotting Fish Guts.

Gross Meter: 🤮🤮🤮🤮

The Romans didn't use ketchup. They used **garum**—a sauce made by **fermenting fish intestines in the sun** until it turned into a liquidy, salty soup of stink. People put it on EVERYTHING: meat, veggies, even fruit. Imagine the smell of fish left out in a hot car for a week...now imagine pouring that on your salad.

Buon appetito!

2. The Candy That Could Kill You

Gross Meter: 🤮🤮

In Victorian England, colorful candies were all the rage—but the dyes used to color them? **Lead. Mercury. Arsenic.** ☠ One famous case: peppermint candies laced with **arsenic** killed 21 people and poisoned 200 more.

Sweet? Yes.

Safe? Not so much.

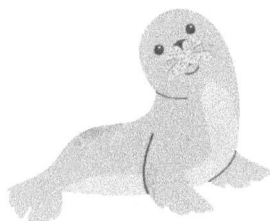

3. Greenland's Bird-in-a-Seal Surprise

Gross Meter: 🤢🤢🤢🤢🤢

Kiviak is a traditional dish made by stuffing a whole seal with **hundreds of tiny birds** (called auks). The seal is then **sewn shut, sealed with fat, and buried underground for months** to ferment. When it's dug up, the birds are soft, juicy, and eaten whole—**feathers, beaks, bones and all**.

Forget chicken nuggets. This is *Seal Surprise Deluxe*.

4. Medieval Jelly Made from Cow Feet

Gross Meter: 🤢🤢

Back in the day, people didn't buy gelatin in little packets. They made it by **boiling animal feet** for hours until the bones and tendons turned into a slimy goop. This goo was strained and used to make jellies, aspics, and wobbly desserts.

So next time you see a shimmering jelly mold, just picture a pot full of **bubbling cow toes**.

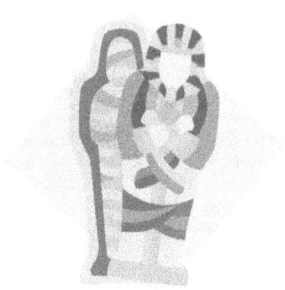

5. Mummy Powder for Medicine (and Maybe Dessert?)

Gross Meter: 💀 💀

During the Renaissance, people believed ground-up mummies had healing powers. So they **dug up real Egyptian mummies**, crushed them into powder, and added it to tonics and food. It was known as **"mumia"**, and some records even suggest it ended up in **sweet treats**.

Yes, people used to eat **dead people.** Let that one sink in.

6. Snail Slime Syrup for Sore Throats

Gross Meter: 🐌 🐌

Snail slime was a hot health trend in the 1600s. People would **mash snails and strain their goo**, mixing it with sugar to create a cough syrup. Sticky. Slimy. Soothing?

Hard pass.

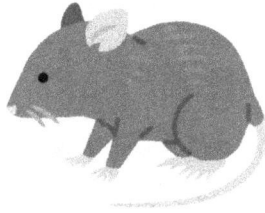

7. Salted Mice on Toast (An Actual Recipe)

Gross Meter:

In Elizabethan England, doctors prescribed **salted, skinned mice on toast** to treat bed-wetting in kids.

No word on whether it worked—but it definitely ruined breakfast.

8. Blood Pudding: It's Not What You Think

Gross Meter:

This traditional dish, still eaten in parts of Europe today, is made from **pig's blood mixed with fat, oats, and spices**, then cooked into a sausage-like loaf.

It's not dessert. It's... breakfast!

WOULD YOU RATHER?

Would you rather eat:
- A fermented bird with feathers
- Or jelly made from cow feet?

Would you rather sip:
- A snail syrup smoothie
- Or arsenic peppermint tea?

Would you rather snack on:
- Mummy powder cookies
- Or salt-crusted mice toast?

GROSS!

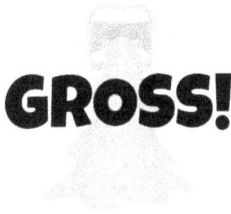

Chapter Recap: Then vs. Yuck

Sure, people didn't have TikTok or pizza delivery 500 years ago... but did they have to **eat birds buried in seals**? Apparently, yes.

They also:

- Thought poison was candy

- Used dead people as medicine

- Made dessert from hooves and goo

So next time you complain about your school lunch, just remember: **at least it's not mouse toast.**

Up next: Things get creepier. We're talking **bugs, brains, and eyeballs on the menu—today.**

Chapter 3

Bugs, Brains & Eyeballs —Oh My!

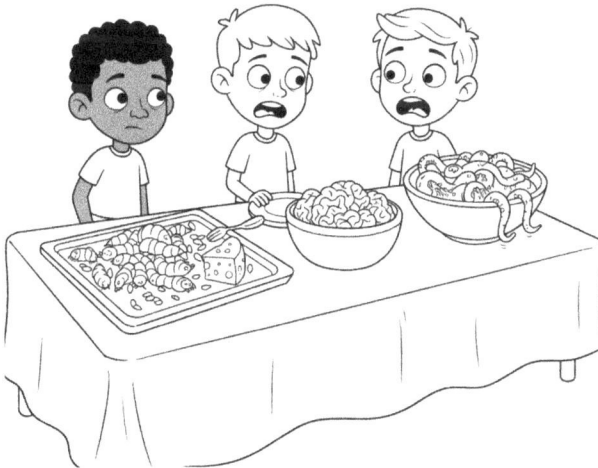

People love to say, "Don't judge a book by its cover." But what about a food that's *still alive*? Or staring back at you?

In this chapter, we're chomping into the world's **weirdest edible creatures**, from maggot cheese to eyeball juice.

~

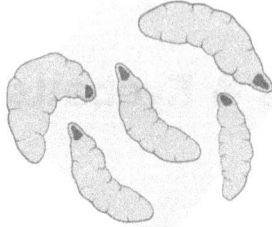

1. Maggot Cheese from Sardinia

Gross Meter: 🤢🤢🤢🤢🤢

Say cheese! Or don't.

Casu marzu is a traditional cheese from Sardinia (an island in Italy) that's famous for one thing: **it's filled with live maggots.**

Yes, really.

The cheese is purposely left out so **flies lay eggs inside it**. When the maggots hatch, they eat the cheese, poop it out, and make it super soft and stinky. **Locals eat it while the maggots are still wriggling.** Some even wear goggles to avoid eye attacks from jumping larvae.

Bon appétit?

2. Deep-Fried Brains—Crispy on the Outside, Squishy on the Inside

Gross Meter: 🧠🧠🧠

In parts of the U.S. (especially the Midwest) and many countries around the world, **animal brains are a delicacy**. Cow brains, pig brains, and even monkey brains are sometimes served grilled, fried, or stewed. They're high in fat, rich in flavor... and have a really, really slimy texture.

Just don't overcook them—**they melt.** 😬

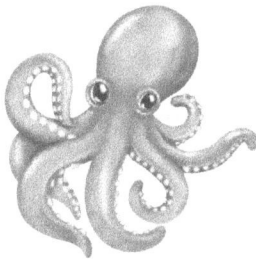

3. Wiggling Octopus Tentacles (Still Moving!)

Gross Meter: 🐙🐙🐙🐙

In Korea, there's a dish called **sannakji**—raw octopus that's chopped up and served **immediately**, while the nerves are still active. That means when you pick up a tentacle with chopsticks, **it moves**. Sometimes, the suction cups still stick to your tongue as you chew.

It's not just creepy—it can be **dangerous** if it sticks in your throat.

4. Balut: A Duck Egg with a Surprise Inside

Gross Meter: 😖😖😖😖

Balut is a **fertilized duck egg**—meaning, yes, a baby duck is *partially developed* inside the egg. It's boiled and eaten whole, feathers and all. You might see tiny bones. Or a little beak. Popular in the Philippines, it's considered a **power snack**.

You just crack it, slurp it, and try not to look too closely. 😬

5. Bug Buffet: Crickets, Worms, and Scorpions, Oh My!

Gross Meter: 😖

Insects are eaten around the world—in fact, over **2 billion people** eat bugs as a regular part of their diet! Popular creepy-crawly snacks:

- **Fried crickets** (Thailand)

- **Mealworm tacos** (Mexico)

- **Scorpion lollipops** (USA novelty treat)

- **Ant eggs** (Colombia)

Fun fact: Bugs are actually high in **protein, fiber, and minerals**.

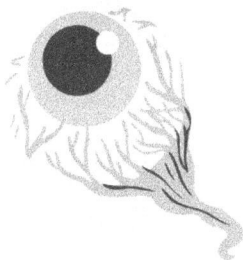

6. Eyeball Soup & Juices

Gross Meter:

In some Mongolian and Chinese traditional dishes, animal eyeballs are added to soups, broths, and even **drinks.** Why? Supposedly they're full of nutrients and believed to help with **eye health.** Sometimes they're served floating in broth like jelly grapes. Sometimes... they burst.

I'll take water, thanks.

7. Snake Wine: Drink With a Bite

Gross Meter:

In Vietnam and parts of China, bottles of **snake wine** are sold as health tonics. It's literally a bottle of **rice wine with a whole snake inside.** Some versions even use **cobra venom**, which is believed to give the drinker energy and power.

Care for a sip? Or are you more of a root beer kind of person?

Pamela Pettyfeather

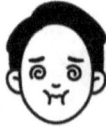

WOULD YOU EAT IT?

TALLY TIME!

Keep track and score yourself. Would you take a bite of...

Food	YES	NO	ARE YOU KIDDING?!
Maggot Cheese	☐	☐	☐
Fried Brain	☐	☐	☐
Wiggly Octopus	☐	☐	☐
Duck Embryo Egg	☐	☐	☐
Crunchy Crickets	☐	☐	☐
Eyeball Juice	☐	☐	☐
Snake Wine	☐	☐	☐

Tally your "YES" answers:

0-2: Gag Reflex Rookie **3-5:** Adventurous Appetizer **6-7:** Fearless Food Freak

GROSS!

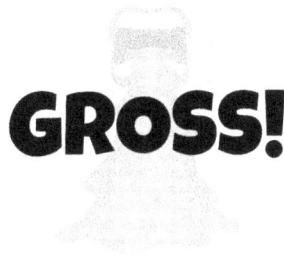

Chapter Recap: What's On the Menu?

Here's what people eat *right now* in different parts of the world:

- Cheese filled with **live maggots**

- Eggs with **tiny ducks inside**

- Moving tentacles

- Floating eyeballs

- And drinks with **snakes in a bottle**

Remember: Just because it's gross to you doesn't mean it's not someone else's favorite snack.

Next up: What happens *after* the food goes down?

Chapter 4

Your Body on Gross Food

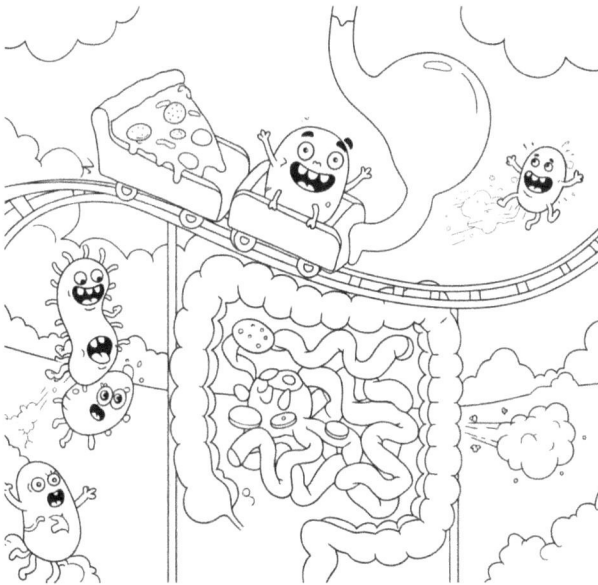

You've swallowed some seriously weird stuff by now—bugs, slime, feet jelly, maybe even a beaver's butt gland. But what happens after that disgusting food goes down your throat? This chapter is all about what happens **inside your body**

when you eat something gross. Spoiler alert: It gets weird. And loud.

And sometimes... explosive.

Let's take the grossness **underground**—right into your gut.

~

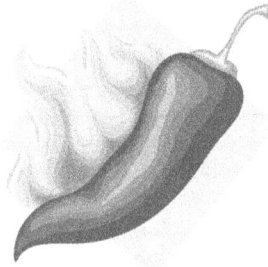

1. Your Brain Thinks Spicy Food Is an Emergency

Gross Meter: 🔥💀

When you eat chili peppers, you're not tasting "heat." You're feeling **pain**. The chemical **capsaicin** tricks your brain into thinking your mouth is **on fire**. That's why your face turns red, you sweat like you just ran a marathon, and your nose starts to run.

Your brain screams: **"ABANDON TONGUE!"**

2. That Gurgling Sound? That's Your Intestines Yelling

Gross Meter:

You know that awkward *blub-blub-groooowl* sound your stomach makes in the middle of class? It's not because you're hungry—it's your **intestines squishing air around** like a giant, wet whoopee cushion.

It's called **borborygmi** (yes, that's a real word), and your body does it all day long. You're basically a walking balloon animal.

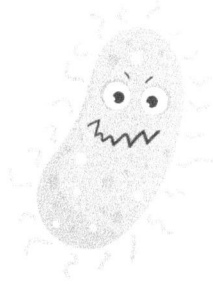

3. Farts Are Made by Hungry Bacteria

Gross Meter:

Your intestines are full of **trillions of bacteria** that help digest your food.

The problem? When they break down certain foods—like beans, broccoli, or dairy—they create **gas**. That gas builds up and exits out the *back door*.

The smell? It comes from tiny amounts of **hydrogen sulfide**—the same gas found in *volcanoes and rotten eggs.*

Congratulations! You're a portable stink machine.

4. Some People Burp Through Their Nose

Gross Meter: ☺

When food or gas pushes back up your throat, it can sneak into your **nasal passages**, especially if you laugh or hiccup while eating. That's how you get the dreaded **nose burp**—a fizzy, acidic, sometimes chewed-up blast right out of your nostrils.

Also known as: **the reverse sneeze of shame.**

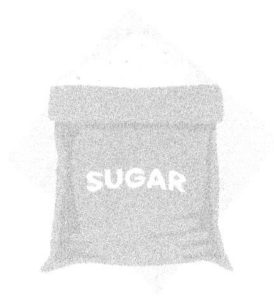

5. Too Much Sugar = Food Hangover

Gross Meter: ☺

Ever eaten way too much Halloween candy and felt dizzy, sweaty, or like the inside of your skull turned into a bounce house? That's called a **sugar crash**. Your blood sugar skyrockets, your body freaks out, and then you suddenly run out of energy like a forgotten phone battery.

Symptoms may include:

- Brain fog

- Belly aches

- Regret

- Crying in your beanbag chair

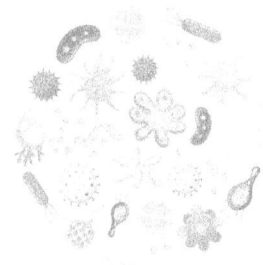

6. Your Gut Is a Bacteria Party (And You're the Host)

Gross Meter: 😝💩

Inside your body right now:

💥 **Over 100 trillion bacteria**

👄 More microbes than **human cells**

🍔 They digest your food, make vitamins... and sometimes cause gas, bloating, or even... poop emergencies.

Some scientists call your gut bacteria a **"second brain"**— but this one mostly thinks about snacks and explosions.

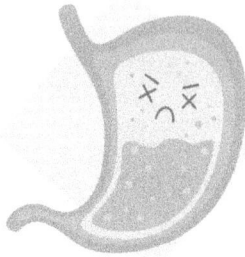

7. Vomit Is Your Body's Emergency Eject Button

Gross Meter: 🤮🤮🤮

When your body detects spoiled, toxic, or disgusting food, it slams the **"NOPE"** button. Muscles contract, your stomach flips, your mouth waters, and **everything you ate launches out the front exit**—fast.

Fun fact: Some animals, like rats, **can't vomit**. That's why they're extra picky eaters.

You, on the other hand? You've got a **built-in barf cannon.**

Gross? Yes.

Miraculous? Also yes.

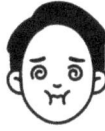

INSIDE OUT DIGESTIVE ADVENTURE

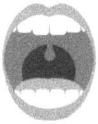

Mouth: Chewed and coated in spit (yum).

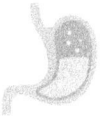

Stomach: Bathed in acid and mushed into sludge.

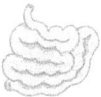

Small Intestine: Sucked dry of nutrients by bacteria.

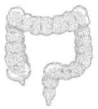

Large Intestine: Soaked like a sponge.

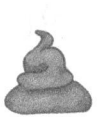

Exit Time: See you later, pizza.

GROSS!

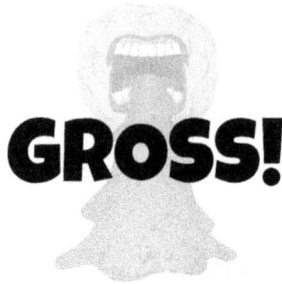

Chapter Recap: You Are a Walking Science Experiment

Your body is a *weird, gooey, noisy machine* that:

- Burps through its nose

- Sweats when it thinks food is fire

- Turns beans into fart bombs

- Builds energy out of pizza sludge

- And knows when to **eject everything** at top speed

You've never been more disgusting—and it's awesome.

Next up: What's that smell?! It might be a fruit that reeks like gym socks... or cheese that smells like your dad's feet.

Chapter 5
Food That Smells Like Trouble

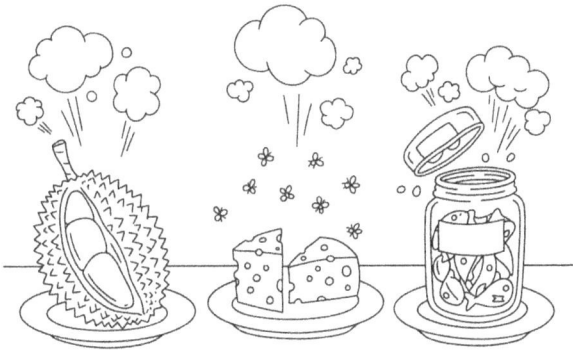

Taste is important. Texture? Big deal. But smell? **Smell is the boss.**

Your nose is your personal food security system—sniffing out anything funky, fishy, or faintly foot-like before you swallow. And trust us... some foods set off ALL the alarms.

Let's sniff our way through the stinkiest, smelliest, most nose-wrecking foods on Earth.

$\sim$

1. Durian: The Fruit That Smells Like Garbage Fire

Gross Meter: 😨😨😨😨

Durian is known as the **"King of Fruits"** in Southeast Asia. It's also known as **"Smells Like Dead Animal in a Sweatsock."** Some people describe it as:

- Rotting onions

- Hot trash juice

- Sweaty gym locker dipped in vanilla

It's banned on buses, trains, and hotels in many countries... but people LOVE the taste once they get past the stench. You just have to survive the first 10 seconds without gagging.

2. Limburger Cheese: Feet, Anyone?

Gross Meter: 😨😨😨

Ever walked into a room and thought, "Did someone take off their shoes and forget them here for 3 weeks?" That's what **Limburger cheese** smells like. And there's a scientific reason: it's made with the **same bacteria found on human skin**—specifically, in sweaty areas like armpits and toes.

Yes, it's *toe cheese*. And people eat it on purpose.

3. Surströmming: The Rotten Fish Can of Doom

Gross Meter: 💀 💀 💀 💀 💀 💀

Straight out of Sweden, **surströmming** is a type of canned fermented herring that's so stinky it's **usually opened outdoors**, and **underwater**, just to keep the smell from attacking bystanders.

The can is often **swollen with gas** from fermentation, and when it's opened? Boom. Rotten eggs + roadkill + sewage = your new least favorite sandwich.

Some people say it's delicious once you stop crying.

4. Truffles: Fancy Fungi That Smell Like Fumes

Gross Meter: 💀 💀

Truffles are a gourmet delicacy, shaved onto pasta or infused into oils. Chefs love them. Rich people love them. But guess what? They smell like:

- Gasoline

- Wet socks

- Wet dog fur left in a car trunk

Some even smell faintly like **old popcorn feet**. Yet they sell for **thousands of dollars per pound**. Proof that being expensive doesn't mean being not-gross.

5. Garlic Breath That Won't Quit

Gross Meter: 🤢

Garlic is delicious. But after you eat it? You don't just *smell* like garlic—you *become* garlic.

Why? The sulfur compounds in garlic **absorb into your bloodstream**, so your lungs literally exhale garlic vapor, and your **sweat starts to smell too.**You can brush, floss, gargle, cry...

The stink is coming from *inside* the house.

6. Cutting Onions = Instant Nose Attack

Gross Meter: 🤢

You know that *onion sting*? That's because cutting onions releases **sulfuric acid gas**, which floats into your eyes and **turns your tears into tiny acid pools**. Your body cries to flush it out.

Basically, onions are **chemical weapons in vegetable form**.

(Delicious weapons, though.)

7. Stinky Tofu: So Wrong, It's Right

Gross Meter: 👃👃👃

This Taiwanese dish is tofu that's been fermented in a mix of **vegetable goo, mold, and sometimes milk or meat juice**. It smells like **rotting garbage soaked in feet water**.

Yet food lovers line up for it because... well, flavor? Bravery? TikTok content?

No one's totally sure.

Smell Check: Fun Nose Factoids!

- Your **taste buds** only detect 5 things (sweet, salty, sour, bitter, umami).

- Your **nose** handles the rest—*about 80% of flavor comes from smell!*

- You can detect over **1 trillion smells**.

- Too bad most of them come from your lunchbox.

- If food **smells like sulfur**, it probably has **rotten eggs, old meat, or broccoli** in it. Yum!

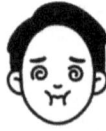

STINK SHOWDOWN

SMELL BATTLE

Which smells worse?

Match-Up   **You Decide!**

Durian vs. Old Onions   _____

Limburger vs. Armpit
Sweat   _____

Surströmming vs. Wet
Dog Truffles   _____

Garlic Breath vs.
Morning Breath   _____

There are no winners. Only survivors.

GROSS!

Chapter Recap: Follow Your Nose

Your nose is trying to help you. Trust it.

This chapter featured:

- Fruit that smells like farts

- Cheese that smells like feet

- Fish that smells like zombie breath

- And tofu that could qualify as chemical warfare

Remember: the stinkiest foods are sometimes the tastiest. Or... the most traumatic.

Up next: What makes some foods **so weird** even scientists scratch their heads? Enter the mad world of **mystery chemicals and flavor fakery.**

Chapter 6

Creepy Chemistry in the Kitchen

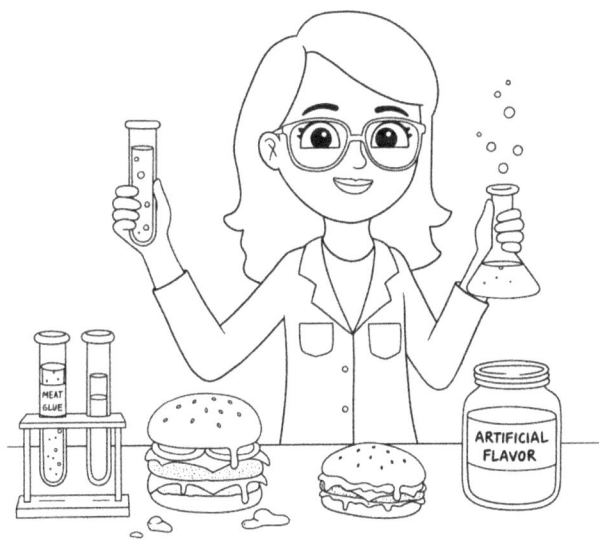

Chemistry is everywhere—even in your lunchbox. That "strawberry" flavor? Probably didn't come from a berry. That steak? Might've been **glued together** like a craft project.

In this chapter, we're exposing the **sneaky science experiments** that make modern food taste, look, and feel... well, **like food.** Sort of.

Let's enter the **kitchen laboratory**. Just don't forget your gloves.

~

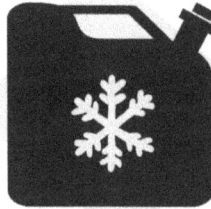

1. Strawberry Flavor... Made with Chemicals from a Beavers' Butt and Antifreeze?

Gross Meter: 💩 🤮

Artificial strawberry flavor can contain up to **50 different chemicals,** many of which are made in a lab. Some come from **petroleum**, and a few are also used in things like:

- Perfume

- Paint thinner

- Antifreeze

And remember our old pal **castoreum**? That beaver butt juice we talked about in Chapter 1? Yeah—it can also be used to boost "natural" strawberry and vanilla flavor.

Suddenly, real strawberries sound pretty good.

2. Meat Glue: Turning Scraps into "Steak"

Gross Meter: 😐🤢

Restaurants and factories often use **transglutaminase**, aka **"meat glue"**, to fuse together tiny scraps of meat and shape them into **perfect-looking steaks**. It's totally legal— and invisible once cooked.

So that fancy filet mignon? Might actually be a **Frankensteak**.

(P.S. It's also used in imitation crab, chicken nuggets, and some lunch meats.)

3. The Truth About Food Dyes

Gross Meter: 🤢

Red 40. Yellow 5. Blue 1. Sounds like a robot team, right?

These are **synthetic food dyes** made from **coal tar** or **petroleum byproducts**—a.k.a. stuff used in car parts and roofing materials. They're used to make:

- Candy

- Sports drinks

- Breakfast cereal

- Rainbow-colored "fruit" snacks

Some dyes are banned in Europe. But in the U.S.? Still totally snack-legal.

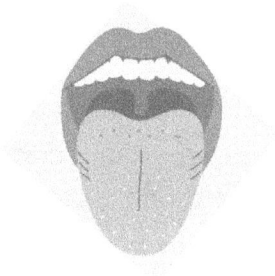

4. Why Artificial Flavors Stick to Your Tongue

Gross Meter: 🫤

Ever wondered why fake cheese dust won't leave your fingers—or your taste buds?

That's **flavor encapsulation**: a technique where scientists **trap tiny flavor molecules in fat or starch bubbles** so they **pop open** as you chew. It makes the taste stronger and longer-lasting. But it also means your tongue is **playing with micro flavor bombs**.

Explosive nachos, anyone?

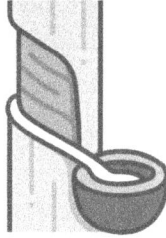

5. Bubble Gum Was Originally Made from Tree Sap and Rubber

Gross Meter: ☺

The first bubble gum was made from **chicle**, a rubbery sap from trees. Later, companies used **synthetic rubber**—yes, like tires—to get that perfect chew. Modern gum still uses plastic-based bases, along with:

- Artificial colors

- Artificial sweeteners

- Artificial *everything*

You're basically chewing a **flavored pink eraser**.

6. Gassed-Up Soda Science

Gross Meter: 😾

That fizzy feeling in soda? It's **carbon dioxide**—the same gas you exhale. But soda also contains **phosphoric acid** (used in rust remover) and sometimes **BVO** (brominated vegetable oil), which was originally developed as a **flame retardant**.

So yeah, it bubbles. But it's kind of a **fireproof burp potion**.

7. The Cheese You Love Might Be a Science Experiment

Gross Meter:

Processed cheese (like in snack slices and nacho sauce) isn't regular cheese—it's **cheese + chemicals + oils + emulsifiers.** Some "cheeses" contain **less than 51% actual cheese.** The rest is:

- Flavorings

- Colorants

- Texture stabilizers

Basically: a **cheese-like product** made in a lab. Melts great. Smells weird.

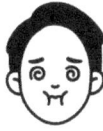

REAL CHEMISTRY OR SCI-FI SNACK?

QUIZ GAME

Which of these is real?

- Cheese made using magnetic microwaves to stretch curds

- Chicken nuggets stuck together with glue

- Gum that changes flavor when you whistle

- Fruit snacks that contain zero fruit

GROSS!

Chapter Recap: Welcome to the Food Lab

Behind that snack you just ate? Science. Lots of it.

In this chapter, you discovered:

- Fake strawberries made with lab fumes

- Steaks made with glue

- Chewing gum made from plastic

- Cheese made with science, not cows

Is it food? Is it magic? Is it a chemistry quiz disguised as lunch?

Yes.

Next up: You won't believe the disasters that happen when food production goes wrong. Think Band-Aids in burgers and pink slime surprise.

Chapter 7
Disgusting Discoveries in Fast Food

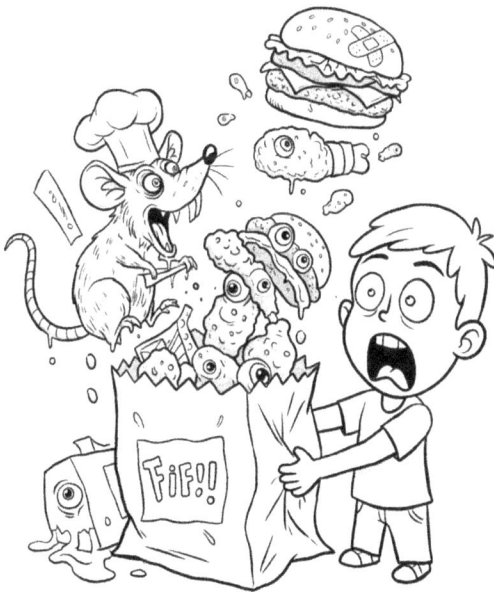

Fast food is fast. It's cheap. It's tasty.

But sometimes... it's also full of **things that should never,**

ever be eaten—like Band-Aids, bleach, or mystery meat paste.

Get ready to unwrap your value meal and find out what might be lurking **under the cheese.**

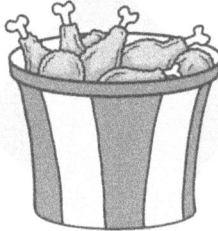

~

1. Fried Lung in a Chicken Bucket

Gross Meter: 🤮🤮

One customer ordered fried chicken... and instead of biting into a juicy dark or white chicken meat, he got a mouthful of **lung** instead.

2. Band-Aid Burger

Gross Meter: 🤮🤮

In 1994, a woman in California bit into a fast-food burger and hit something chewy. Not lettuce. Not cheese. A **used Band-Aid**.

She sued. She got a $5000 in damages. The rest of us got nightmares.

3. Pink Slime: The Secret Inside Some Meat

Gross Meter:

"Pink slime" is a nickname for **lean finely textured beef**—a paste made from beef trimmings, connective tissue, and **ammonia gas**. It's used to bulk up burgers and nuggets. It looks like strawberry yogurt. It's... not. It's banned in some countries. In the U.S., it's still legal.

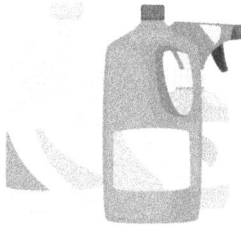

4. Cleaning Chemicals Don't Cleanse Your Palate

Gross Meter:

Fast food kitchens use **powerful cleaning chemicals** to scrub down equipment. Sometimes those chemicals accidentally end up **in the food**. There've been multiple reports of:

- Bleach in burritos

- Sanitizer in smoothies

- Disinfectant nuggets

Side effects: Burning throats, vomiting, emergency room visits... and probably switching to home-packed lunches.

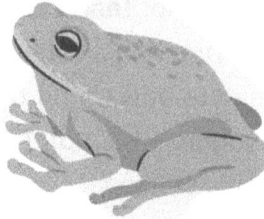

5. Frog in the Salad

Gross Meter: 😩🤢

Multiple customers at major chains have opened their salads to find a **frog** staring back. In one case, it was still **alive**.

6. Tooth in the Fries, Dental Filling in the Burger

Gross Meter: 🤮🤮

At a fast food chain in Japan, a customer bit into her burger and crunched down on something hard. It turned out to be **dental material**—as in, part of a **filling**. Another fast food fan found a **human tooth in their fries**!

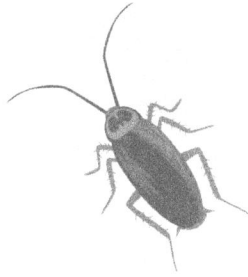

7. Cockroaches & Rats in Your Soup

Gross Meter: ✶ ☺ ☺ ☺

A customer eating at the popular chain discovered what looked like part of a **cockroach** in their beef bowl. This wasn't even the first bug-related incident—just months earlier, a **dead rat** was found in a bowl of miso soup.

The chain responded by temporarily **shutting down nearly all their restaurants**. When your food sends customers screaming *and* health inspectors running?

Not ideal.

Real Headlines, Real Nightmares

All of the above incidents were **reported in the news**, which means these weren't just urban legends. People have *actually*:

- Chomped Band-Aids

- Discovered frogs

- Eaten ammonia-treated meat

- Bit into **plastic gloves, hairballs, and even bullets** (yep—Google it)

And yet... we keep going back. Why? **Because fries.**

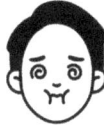

FACTORY FAIL!

REPORTING FORM

Help us report the next fast food disaster! Fill in the blanks:

I ordered a: _____

But instead I got: _____

It tasted like: _____

My reaction was:
- ☐ Screamed
- ☐ Vomited
- ☐ Took a picture
- ☐ Ate it anyway

GROSS!

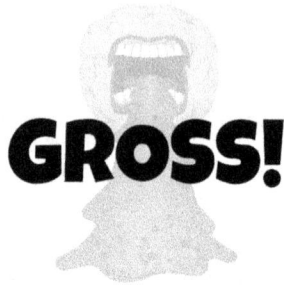

Chapter Recap: Extra Gross, No Extra Charge

Fast food can be fun. But it can also include:

- Rats

- Chemicals

- Band-Aids

- Body parts

- Surprise frogs

Next time you unwrap your burger, just hope it's ketchup— not **something from someone's sock drawer.**

Coming up: You've made it through bugs, body parts, and barf science. But what about your **favorite treats**? Get ready to ruin dessert.

Chapter 8

Gross Candy, Grosser Origins

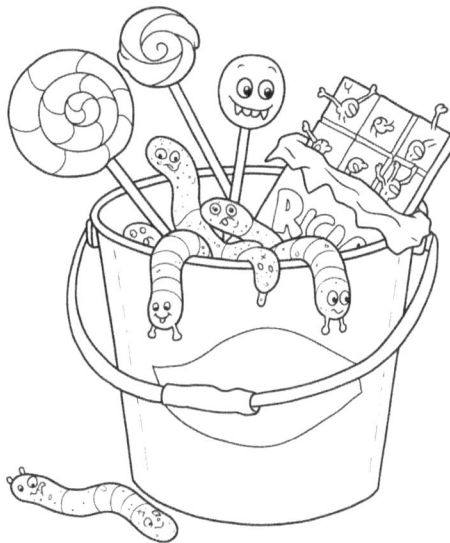

Candy is colorful. Candy is chewy. Candy is fun. But... candy is also **disgusting.**

From insect parts to animal bones to sneaky chemicals, some of the world's sweetest treats have the **grossest backstories**.

Get ready to never look at your gummy bear the same way again!

~

1. Red Candy = Crushed Bugs

Gross Meter: 🪲🪲

That shiny red color in jelly beans, popsicles, and strawberry candy? It often comes from **cochineal**—tiny beetles crushed into powder to make **carmine dye**.

Yup. Your fruit snacks are **bug-flavored**. With extra crunch. (Spoiler: We also mentioned this in Chapter 1, but candy deserves its own special horror story.)

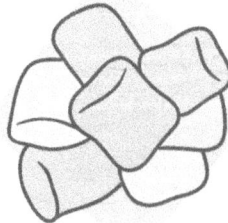

2. Marshmallows Are Made of Bones and Skin

Gross Meter: 😬😬

Marshmallows get that squish from **gelatin**—a jelly-like substance made by **boiling pig and cow bones, skin, and tendons.** It's also what gives Jell-O that jiggle and jelly beans that chew. Basically, you're eating **bone goo** mixed with tons of sugar.

Tasty!

3. Chocolate Can Legally Contain Insect Parts

Gross Meter: 🤢🤢🤢

According to the FDA, chocolate is allowed to contain up to **60 insect fragments per 100 grams**. Why? Because bugs are **everywhere**, and it's impossible to keep them all out during harvesting and production.

So that rich, creamy candy bar? It might include a little extra *crunch*—from **beetles, ants, or fly legs.**

Sweet.

4. Sour Candy Can Burn Holes in Your Tongue

Gross Meter: 🤢

Ever eaten so many Warheads or sour gummies that your tongue felt like a battlefield? That's because super-sour candy contains **citric acid**—the same stuff used in **cleaning products**. In large amounts, it can:

- Peel off layers of your tongue

- Cause tiny burns and ulcers

- Make you talk funny for days

Some kids have even **blistered their mouths** trying to win sour-eating contests.

5. Cotton Candy: Invented by a Dentist

Gross Meter: 😖

Yes, you read that right.

The inventor of cotton candy was **William Morrison**, a dentist. He spun sugar into floss-like threads and called it "Fairy Floss." He also probably made a **fortune fixing cavities** caused by his own invention.

Business strategy: *10/10, morally questionable.*

6. Halloween Candy Used to Contain Poison (On Purpose!)

Gross Meter: ☠️

In the 1800s, candy makers used **toxic metals like lead, arsenic, and mercury** to create bright colors. Green gumdrops? Might have contained **copper sulfate.** Red candies? Sometimes **vermilion, made from mercury.**

Kids died. Laws were made. And we're still eating weird stuff. Just less *immediately* deadly now.

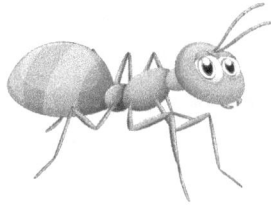

7. Insect Candy Is Now a Trend (and a Dare)

Gross Meter: 🤢🤢

Want a lollipop with a real scorpion inside? How about chocolate-covered ants? Jelly beans with cricket legs?

These exist. You can buy them. Some kids think they're hilarious. Others think they're **revenge candy from the bug kingdom.**

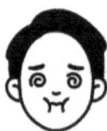

CANDY OR CURSED?

QUIZ GAME

Which of these is real?

- Licorice root can mess with your heart rhythm.

- Bubble gum used to contain whale fat.

- Some candies are coated in shellac —a shiny finish made from bugs.

- Caramel was once used as shoe polish.

GROSS!

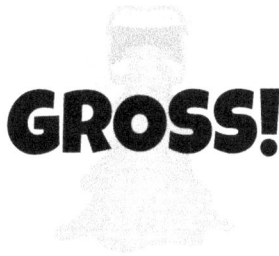

Chapter Recap: Trick or Treat... or Trauma?

In this chapter, you discovered:

- Candy colored with crushed beetles

- Gummies made from animal bones

- Chocolate that legally contains bugs

- Sour stuff that **burns your mouth off**

- And dentists who invented sugar bombs

Still hungry?

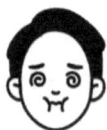

FINAL GROSS METER

HOW GROSSED OUT ARE YOU NOW?

Score	Level
0-5 facts that made you gag	Mildly Moldy
6-15 facts	Certified Snack Skeptic
16-25 facts	Fearless Food Freak
26+ facts	You Need a Stomach of Steel (and Maybe Therapy)

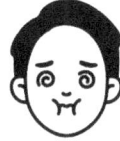

CONCLUSION: Now You Know. Sorry About That

Whew.

You made it.

You survived bugs in your chocolate.

Bones in your gummies.

Farts in your intestines.

And band-aids in your burger.

You now know:

- What pink slime is

- How many bug bits are legal in candy

- Why your own body is basically a burping, farting bacteria hotel

- And that ancient people used to eat **mummified humans on purpose**

So, yeah. You're officially a **Certified Gross Food Genius.**

Next time someone bites into a bright red cupcake and says, "Mmm, so good!" You can smile and say, "You know that's made of beetles, right?"

Knowledge is power.

Gross knowledge is better.

Stay curious. Stay weird. Stay disgustingly awesome.

And please—don't read this book while eating.

FREE & FUN STUFF!

Want More Gross Fun?

Did you love this weird, wacky, and slightly stomach-turning journey through the world of gross food?

Good news: **you've unlocked some truly disgusting bonuses** (in the best way possible):

Get the FREE Audiobook

Listen to *Weird Facts About Food (Gross.)* on the go— perfect for road trips, classrooms, or brushing your teeth while gagging over gummy bear bones.

Download the Bonus Activity Pack

Includes a **word search**, **crossword puzzle**, and **coloring pages** inspired by the grossest facts in the book.

🖋 Join the Weird Facts Family Club

When you sign up, you'll get:

• Early access to future *Weird Facts* books

• Invitations to help us pick the next book's topic

• A chance to share your own favorite weird facts!

Ready to grab your free bonuses and join the weirdest club on the internet?

Scan the QR code below or visit: www.pettyfeatherpublishing.com/weirdfactsbonus

See you in the slime zone!

—Pamela & the Pettyfeather Family

Also by Pamela Pettyfeather

Books for Curious & Clever Kids Series

Global Explorations. Bold Questions. Awesome Holidays.

Welcome to the Books for Curious & Clever Kids series—a collection of lively nonfiction books that bring world traditions, history, and culture to life for kids ages 8–12!

These books are designed for the endlessly curious and the slightly-too-clever kids who always ask:

"Wait... why do we do that?"

"Where did that come from?"

"And what do other people do today?!"

Each book in the series explores a major holiday or tradition through, Global stories and celebrations, fun facts and surprising history and Kid-friendly recipes, activities, and fun.

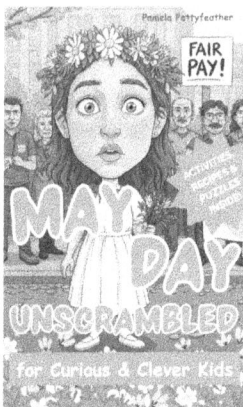

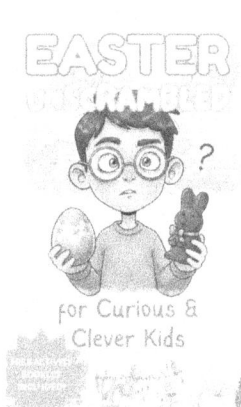

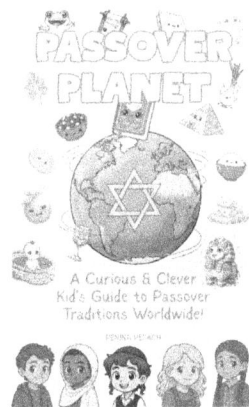

Easter Unscrambled for Curious & Clever Kids

Why do we hunt for eggs on Easter? Where did the Easter Bunny come from? And what do ancient gods and chocolate bunnies have in common? **Easter Unscrambled** is the perfect blend of fascinating facts and hands-on fun — ideal for kids ages 7-12 who love puzzles, history, and surprises. This interactive book takes readers on a 4,000-year adventure through the origins of Easter — from ancient gods and springtime festivals to Easter egg hunts and chocolate bunnies.

$\sim$

Passover Planet: A Curious & Clever Kids' Guide to Passover Traditions Worldwide!

Frogs. Pharaohs. Pancakes. Passover Like You've Never Seen It Before! Get ready to travel through **3,000 years of Passover celebrations**—from **ancient Egypt to modern space stations**, from Moroccan mimouna feasts to Ecuadorian chocolate charoset! In **Passover Planet**, kids will **1)** Discover global Passover traditions from **Ethiopia, Persia, Poland, Iraq, South America** & more **2)** Learn about cool customs like scallion fights and Afikoman ransoms **3)** Explore **Seders with matzah pizza**, spicy charoset, and teff flatbread...

$\sim$

May Day Unscrambled for Curious & Clever Kids

Why do people dance around poles in spring... while others wave protest signs? From leafy legends to labor marches, **May Day Unscrambled** unravels one of the world's most surprising holidays!

Kids will travel through time and across the globe as they explore: 1) **Ancient spring festivals** like Beltane and Walpurgisnacht **2) British traditions like maypole dancing and the May Queen** 3) The rise of **International Workers' Day** and the fight for fair labor and 4) Global May Day celebrations in **France, Finland, Hawaii**, and more!

Halloween Unscrambled and *Christmas Unscrambled* coming soon...

∾

Scan the QR code below for more about this series

Quiz Answers

Chapter 1

1-B, 2-A, 3-E, 4-D, 5-C

Chapter 6

1 = Fake (for now)
2 = Real (meat glue!)
3 = Fake (but fun idea)
4 = VERY real

Chapter 8

1 = ☑ Real
2 = ✗ Fake (but fun)
3 = ☑ Real (shellac comes from the lac bug!)
4 = ✗ But now you're imagining it, aren't you?

www.ingramcontent.com/pod-product-compliance
Lightning Source LLC
Chambersburg PA
CBHW062026040426
42447CB00010B/2162